Urinary tract infection

The comprehensive guide on Urinary tract infection in both men and women

By Linda J. Franklin

TABLE OF CONTEXT

Chapter 1: Urinary tract infection

UTIs are characterized as difficult or uncomplicated clinically. Uncomplicated UTIs, also known as cystitis and upper UTIs, often afflict people who are otherwise healthy and do not have structural or neurological abnormalities of the urinary system (pyelonephritis). Women, previous UTIs, sexual activity, vaginal infections, diabetes, obesity, and a family history of the condition are among the risk factors for cystitis. According to definitions, complicated UTIs are those that are linked to conditions that weaken the immune system or host defense, such as urinary obstruction, urinary retention brought on by neurological conditions, immunosuppression, renal failure, renal transplantation, pregnancy, and the presence of foreign objects like calculi, indwelling catheters, or other drainage devices. Indwelling catheters are to blame for 70–80% of complex UTIs in the US, or 1 million infections annually, according to research. The majority of secondary bloodstream infections are caused by catheter-associated UTIs (CAUTIs), which are also linked to higher rates of morbidity and death. Long-term catheterization, being a woman, being older, and having diabetes are risk factors for getting a CAUTIs

Both Gram-positive and Gram-negative bacteria, as well as certain fungi, may result in UTIs. Uropathogenic Escherichia coli is the most typical causal agent for both simple and complex UTIs (UPEC). Klebsiella pneumonia, Staphylococcus saprophyticus, Enterococcus faecalis, group B streptococcus (GBS), Proteus mirabilis, Pseudomonas aeruginosa, Staphylococcus aureus, and Candida are the next most common bacteria associated with uncomplicated UTIs after UPEC. Enterococcus spp., K. pneumoniae, Candida spp., S. aureus, P. mirabilis, P. aeruginosa, and GBS9 are the most prevalent causal agents for complex UTIs, with UPEC being second-most prevalent.

Antibiotics are often prescribed to patients who have symptoms of a UTI; however, these medications have the potential to permanently change the natural microbiota of the vagina and gastrointestinal tract and to foster the growth of bacteria that are resistant to a variety of antibiotics. The potential for multidrug-resistant uropathogens to colonize spaces that the changed microbiota no longer fills may be a concern. Importantly, the "golden age" of antibiotics is passing, and as a result, there is a growing demand for therapies that are logically developed and non-toxic. Uropathogens from the urine of women with symptomatic UTIs has been directly analyzed in recent investigations using RNA sequencing. We now know the molecular specifics of how uropathogens adhere, colonize, and adapt to the nutritionally restricted bladder environment, avoid immune monitoring, and survive and spread in the urinary system thanks to this research, fundamental science, and better animal models.

A urinary tract infection is quite likely to occur in a woman. One in two-lifetime chances are given by some specialists, with many women experiencing recurrent infections for years on end. In their lifetime, around one in ten men will get a UTI.

The symptoms of a UTI can include:

a scorching sensation when you urinate
a persistent or strong need to urinate, even when it produces little urine when you do
Pee that is black, red, cloudy, or has an odd scent
feeling drained or unsteady
chills or a fever (a sign that the infection may have reached your kidneys)
back or lower abdomen pressure or pain

Different UTIs
Different areas of your urinary system are susceptible to infection. Based on its location, each variety has a unique name.

Bladder cystitis: You may have frequent urination or discomfort when urinating. Along with lower stomach discomfort, you may also have murky or red urine.
Pyelonephritis (kidney): This may result in a fever, chills, nausea, vomiting, and upper back or side discomfort.

Urethritis (urethra): This condition may make you urinate with a discharge and burning.

Reasons for UTIs
Doctors advise women to wipe after using the restroom from front to back in large part due to UTIs. Near the anus lies the urethra, the tube that carries urine from the bladder to the exterior of the body. Sometimes, bacteria from the large intestine, including E. coli, might escape from your anus and enter your urethra. They may then ascend to your bladder and, if the infection is not treated, progress to infect your kidneys. Compared to males, women's urethras are shorter. Bacteria may enter their bladders more easily as a result. Additionally, having sex may spread germs throughout your urinary system.

Due to their genetic makeup, certain women are more prone to developing UTIs. Others are more susceptible to getting infected because of the form of their urinary systems. Due to their compromised immune systems and decreased ability to fight off infections, women with diabetes may be more vulnerable. Multiple sclerosis, hormonal changes, and illnesses that impair urine flow, such as kidney stones, strokes, and spinal cord injuries, are other disorders that might increase your .

Chapter 2: Treatment for urinary tract infection

The most frequent therapy for urinary tract infections is antibiotics if your doctor feels you need them. Always remember to take the whole recommended dosage of medication, even if you begin to feel better. To assist remove the germs from your body, drink a lot of water. To relieve your discomfort.

Cranberry juice is often touted as a treatment or preventative for UTIs. The tannin in the red berry may prevent E. coli bacteria, the most frequent cause of urinary tract infections, from adhering to the walls of your bladder, where they may spread illness. But the study hasn't shown that it significantly lowers infections.

Additionally, experts are researching novel vaccinations, immune system boosters, and hormone replacement therapy for postmenopausal women as potential treatments and preventative measures for UTIs.

long-term UTIs

A UTI in a guy increases his risk of developing another one. One in five women will get a second UTI, and some may experience recurrent UTIs. Most of the time, a unique kind or strain of bacteria causes each illness. However, certain bacteria may enter the cells of your body and grow there, becoming an antibiotic-resistant bacterial colony. They then exit the cells and return to the urinary system.

Treatment for Chronic UTI

Request a treatment plan from your doctor if you have three or more UTIs each year. Taking: is one choice among several.

a little amount of antibiotic is given over a longer length of time to help avoid recurrent infections

After intercourse, which is a typical infection trigger, one dosage of an antibiotic

If symptoms develop, take an antibiotic for a day or two.

a preventative measure without antibiotics

You may determine if you need to contact your doctor by using at-home urine tests, which are available without a prescription. If you are taking antibiotics for a UTI, you may do a test to determine if the infection has been treated (although you still need to finish your prescription). t.

How to Prevent Reinfection of UTIs
You may prevent having another UTI by heeding the advice below:

As soon as you feel the need to urinate, empty your bladder often; don't hurry, and make sure you've emptied it.
Following a bathroom visit, wipe the area from front to back.
Take in a lot of water.
Prefer showers over baths.
Sprays for feminine hygiene, scented douches, and scented bath products should all be avoided since they simply serve to exacerbate discomfort.
Before having intercourse, clean your genitalia.
After intercourse, urinate to clear your urethra of any germs that may have gotten inside.

You may wish to switch to a different technique if you currently use a diaphragm, non-lubricated condoms, or spermicidal jelly. While spermicides and unlubricated condoms might aggravate your urinary system, diaphragms can accelerate the development of germs. Each of these may increase the likelihood of UTI symptoms.

Wear cotton underwear and baggy clothing to keep your genital region dry. Avoid donning nylon underwear and tight jeans.

Chapter 3:Bacteria that causes UTIS

Gram-negative bacteria and gram-positive bacteria are the two major groups of bacteria that cause UTIs.

In contrast to gram-positive bacteria, gram-negative ones have an outer cell membrane. To identify the kind of bacteria when examined under a microscope, a simple test using a violet color dye (known as gram stain) is utilized. The gram-negative bacteria are those that have a membrane that prevents them from being stained by the gram stain and keeps them pink. While gram-negative bacteria have a membrane, gram-positive bacteria do not. As a result, they may readily bind to the dye and look violet under a microscope.

Infections brought on by gram-negative bacteria are more challenging to cure because of this membrane. Additionally, gram-negative bacteria are more harmful to the host than gram-positive bacteria and have enhanced resistance to antibiotics.

Infections in the urinary tract are often brought on by gram-negative bacteria, such as:

Most occurrences of straightforward cystitis and pyelonephritis are caused by Escherichia coli (or E. coli).

Bloodstream infections caused by Klebsiella pneumonia are well-known.

UTIs picked up in hospitals are often caused by Pseudomonas aeruginosa, which may potentially cause deadly sepsis.

The extended-spectrum beta-lactamases (ESBL) enzyme-producing subgroup of gram-negative bacteria is particularly noteworthy. Most beta-lactam antibiotics, such as penicillins, cephalosporins, and monobactam aztreonam, are susceptible to the bacterium, but this enzyme enables the bacteria to resist them. It is unfortunately exceedingly difficult to cure infections caused by ESBL-producing microbes. A few E. coli and Klebsiella pneumonia strains are the most frequent ESBL-producing bacteria. An ESBL-producing bacterium may spread more easily among patients in healthcare facilities or nursing homes.

These are a few instances of gram-positive bacteria that might result in UTI:

Aspergillus saprophyticus
Streptococcus GB
Aerococcus
Enterococcus
Who contracts what bacteria?
We must remember that various patients (children, young women, pregnant women, men, or the elderly) are not equally vulnerable to each kind of UTI bacteria when we examine these patients' susceptibilities. Furthermore, the bacteria that are most likely to be to blame will depend on how you got your UTI (for example, through bladder stones or a catheter in a medical environment). In addition, the urinary tract may become infected by many pathogens at once in certain circumstances; this condition is known as a "polymicrobial infection" in the medical community. Additionally, a few bacteria may colonize a bladder without ever leading to a UTI.

E. coli UTI

When a young, sexually active, non-pregnant woman has an uncomplicated UTI, E. coli bacteria are most often identified in the urinary tract in 75%–80% of cases. This gram-negative bacteria is susceptible to building up a drug resistance.

Our lower intestines are home to a large population of E. coli, which means that human feces may include this organism. While E. coli in your intestines are safe and even beneficial (they help produce vitamin K), they have the potential to be quite harmful when they aren't handled properly.

E. coli may, unfortunately, rather easily go from your anus to your vagina and urethra to produce a UTI. E. coli is sometimes referred to as an opportunistic microbe because of this.

Opportunistic bacteria take advantage of conditions where they would not ordinarily be able to flourish, such as a host with a compromised immune system or a disturbed microbiota (such as the microbiota in the gut or the vagina). In these conditions, they may quickly multiply.

Because of this, you'll be more vulnerable to an assault by an opportunistic bacterium if your vaginal or intestinal flora is out of balance. As opposed to this, the bacteria won't have an opportunity to expand out of control when your microbiome is in a condition of healthy balance.

the miraculous Proteus
A long-term catheter user is more likely to contract the gram-negative bacteria Proteus mirabilis. Due to Proteus mirabilis' capacity to create biofilms and evolve medication resistance, catheter-associated urinary tract infections (CAUTI) are very challenging to treat. The mucosal layer of the urethra may be harmed during catheter insertion, disrupting the natural barrier and promoting bacterial colonization. Furthermore, the catheter tube acts as a highway for bacteria, enabling them to enter the bladder and develop biofilm colonies on its surface.

Hazardous, symptomless bacteriuria, which may result in a potentially fatal urosepsis, can also be brought on by this bacterium in addition to a usual UTI. This is particularly true for older people and those with type-2 diabetes. Urinary stones may also develop as a result of P. mirabilis infections.

The gastrointestinal system often contains P.mirabilis, but little is known about how these bacteria interact with the gut microbiome. Ascending from the gastrointestinal tract to the urine tract is how P.mirabilis are thought to reach the urinary system, however, this is unclear. Indeed, some clinical investigations suggest that this virus may spread from person to person, particularly in a hospital environment. Evidence showing that some P. mirabilis UTI patients have the same strain of P. mirabilis in their feces while other patients have no P. mirabilis in their stools supports this claim.

Staph aureus Pseudomonas
A gram-negative bacteria called P. aeruginosa is one of the ones that cause infections and

urinary tract infections (UTIs) linked with catheters most often in individuals who are immunocompromised. Nevertheless, P. aeruginosa is one of the least studied bacteria, which means that hospitals lack knowledge about how to stop and cure infections brought on by these microbes. Unfortunately, UTIs caused by P. aeruginosa are notoriously difficult to cure. This bacteria not only has several virulent defenses that enable it to survive and distribute antibiotics, but it also swiftly creates biofilms on catheter surfaces to further protect itself from their effects.

pneumonia-causing klebsiella

Particularly recognized for producing sepsis and urinary tract infections (UTI) in neonates as well as adult patients' hospital-acquired UTIs, Klebsiella pneumoniae (K. pneumoniae) is a kind of bacteria. Antibiotic resistance, notably to drugs called carbapenems, is another prominent trait of this gram-negative bacteria.

Humans normally harbor the K. pneumoniae bacterium, although the frequency with which this bacterium is discovered varies depending on several circumstances. For instance, in certain regions of the globe as well as in a hospital context, carrier rates of K. pneumoniae in the population are much higher. Patients who are Asian in ethnicity are more likely to have this bacteria colonize their intestines.

Aspergillus saprophyticus
Gram-positive Staphylococcus saprophyticus (or S. saprophyticus) bacteria are the origin of 10-15% of UTI cases. Young, sexually active women are at risk for 40% of S. saprophyticus UTIs.

The bacterium S. saprophyticus has several highly peculiar traits, however, it has many clinical traits with an E. coli-caused urinary tract infection. For instance, in the late summer and early autumn, they are often discovered in the urinary system of mostly young girls and women. This bacterium causes UTIs in post-menopausal women infrequently, and in the winter and spring, it is less common.

Despite the rarity of S. saprophyticus infection in men, it may strike elderly or ill men.

The good news is that S. saprophyticus UTI seldom results in bacteremia (blood infection) and is typically responsive to most medications, including penicillin.

Aspergillus aureus

S. aureus UTI, unlike S. saprophyticus, often affects pregnant women and those using a urinary catheter. Furthermore, most S. aureus superstrains are resistant to methicillin.

Enterococci

Gram-positive, lactic acid bacteria called enterococci may grow and thrive in the absence or presence of oxygen, and they can withstand temperatures of 4.6 to 9 pH and temperatures between 10 and 45 °C. With enterococci accounting for between 15 and 30 percent of CAUTIs, a urinary catheter is a significant risk factor. Additionally, enterococci rank as the third most common source of UTIs in healthcare facilities.

Diabetes patients are more likely to develop enterococcal UTIs due to their weakened immune systems and inadequate bladder emptying. About 10% of diabetic men have prostate irritation caused by these bacteria, which may also travel to the circulation.

Sadly, antibiotic resistance is increasing among enterococcal superstrains. Since E. faecalis develops tough biofilms, in particular, it is notoriously difficult for medicines to get through these films and eradicate the superbug.

Group B Streptococcus-related Urinary Tract Infection

GBS is a gram-positive chain-forming bacteria that often live in the female reproductive system and lower stomach without presenting any symptoms. According to statistics, just 1% to 2% of UTIs are brought on by the bug.

The two biggest risks for getting a UTI caused by this bacteria are advanced age and pregnancy. In actuality, GBS UTIs may be lethal in older patients. There are extra risk factors for developing a GBS UTI in people with weakened immune systems, such as those with cancer, diabetes, or pre-existing urinary tract abnormalities such as chronic kidney disease or kidney stones.

Although GBS often doesn't manifest any symptoms in females during pregnancy, its presence in the urine or the vagina might offer major risks to the mother and the fetus. Most critically, the infection might enter the child's system during labor and delivery, which can be fatal, if there is a GBS transfer from the mother to the infant. The Centers for Disease Control suggest that all pregnant women be screened at 35–37 weeks due to the significant risk of GBS problems in the unborn child. During labor and delivery, preventative IV antibiotics are advised if a woman tests positive for GBS.

UTI brought on by many disease-causing germs (Polymicrobial UTI)
A UTI with many bacterial types is referred to as polymicrobial. Hospitals are a common source of polymicrobial UTIs, and urinary catheter use is more commonly linked to these infections. Compared to monomicrobial infections, polymicrobial infections are more often linked with Pseudomonas aeruginosa,

whereas monomicrobial infections are more frequently associated with Escherichia coli.

groupings at risk:

the elderly
Individuals with impaired immune systems, such as those with HIV infection, diabetes, or cancer
Various Rare and Emerging UTI Bugs
Aerococcus is a gram-positive cluster-forming microbe that, if left untreated, may result in a potentially fatal bladder, kidney, and blood infection.
A gram-positive bacteria called Corynebacterium urealyticum may lead to the development of large kidney stones as well as chronic inflammation of the bladder and kidneys.
Actinobaculum schaalii: A potentially gram-positive pathogen that is resistant to the first-line antibiotics used to treat UTIs.
Gardnerella vaginalis, which is common in BV-afflicted women and may infect the kidneys and bladder.

several examinations for various microorganisms

Chapter 4: Urinary tract infection in men

Men's Urinary Tract Infections: Signs, Tests, and Treatment

Men may have urinary tract infections (UTIs), even though women often suffer the most from their annoying symptoms. The likelihood of obtaining one increases with age.

abstract urinal artwork

Men will have UTI symptoms at least once throughout their lifetimes, accounting for 13% of all males.

According to the National Institute of Diabetes and Digestive and Kidney Diseases , urinary tract infections (UTIs) are more common in women than in men, with at least 40 to 60 percent of women experiencing a UTI at some point in their lives. However, men are also susceptible to these frequently uncomfortable and potentially harmful infections.

Twelve percent of males will get at least one UTI over their lifetime, according to the

American Urological Association. Furthermore, although urinary tract infections are uncommon in young men, the risk of infection rises with age, with UTIs being more prevalent in men over 50.

Due to simple anatomy, women are more likely to have urinary tract infections: It takes little distance for the bladder to get infected by the pelvic region-specific bacteria that are the main cause of this kind of illness.

The male anatomy, on the other hand, may assist in warding off this kind of illness. For germs to go that far without being washed out or eliminated by the immune system, the longer urethra in males makes this more challenging.

The Risk Factors for UTIs in Men
Males are more likely to get a UTI than females due to several other variables, in addition to age, such as:

increased prostate size
a kidney stone
Diabetes

catheterization of the bladder

Immune system-compromising illness of any kind

Anal sex without protection

Identification of Men's UTI Symptoms

With a urinary tract infection, which often involves an inflammation of the bladder (cystitis), may also include an infection of the lower or upper urinary tract, and — in more severe instances — the kidneys, some individuals may not have any symptoms. Moreover, not every man, woman, or a kid who develops a UTI displays the classic UTI symptoms, although the majority do show at least one or more infection-related symptoms. Furthermore, males seldom get UTIs, and when they do, the symptoms are often not all that dissimilar from those that affect women. Here are some typical UTI signs:

Urinating often
an intense need to urinate that never goes away
urinal release is limited to modest volumes at a time
Urine that is murky, red, or smells unpleasant

lower-abdominal) discomfort in the suprapubic area
Urination that causes burning or anguish
Lower back discomfort, a fever, nausea, or chills together with any of these symptoms may be signs of a kidney infection, a dangerous condition that requires immediate medical attention.

Men's UTI Diagnosis Procedure
A urinary tract infection develops when bacteria (or, less often, a virus or even a fungus) invade the urinary system. 80 to 90 percent of UTI infections, according to the National Kidney Foundation, are caused by one specific bacterium, E. coli.

In the beginning, a urine culture is used to diagnose a urinary tract infection in males just as it does in women. But since a UTI in a guy is often thought to be difficult, further testing is generally required to figure out how it happened.

"This typically includes a CT [computerized tomography] scan to evaluate for kidney stones or other anatomic abnormalities that may be causing this, as well as a special study to determine how much urine he leaves behind after urinating," he says. "This typically includes not only a urinary culture to confirm an infection, but also a special study to determine how much urine he leaves behind after urinating."

It may be important to do further testing if a man exhibits UTI-like symptoms without a positive urine culture, recurring infections, infections caused by the same organism, or both.

Treatment for Men's Urinary Tract Infections
The same course of antibiotics is given to both men and women who have infections to eradicate the bacterium and alleviate UTI symptoms. A woman usually has to take an antibiotic for one to three days if she has an uncomplicated illness. Trost advises that males

should take antibiotics for a longer period—at least seven days.

Men's Urinary Tract Infection Prevention
Trost believes that there isn't anything that younger guys can do to avoid a UTI. Older men, however, may reduce their risk by taking a few measures. One of the best ways to prevent UTIs is to fully empty your bladder each time you pee. It's also crucial to consume enough fluids, particularly water, each day. If you already have a UTI, drinking enough fluids will help flush the germs from the urinary system, which, in some very mild instances, may be sufficient to cure the condition. However, it's still crucial to see your doctor for a diagnosis and recommended course of action if you have any of the UTI symptoms.

Without effective UTI treatment, the infection may swiftly spread and pose a significant, and sometimes deadly, danger. As a result, don't ignore signs like frequent urination or a burning sensation while urinating, and don't believe that you can't have a UTI simply because you're a guy. You should see a doctor right away for a quick examination of these symptoms as well.

Males' STD symptoms vs UTI symptoms
having a sexual activity (whether it be vaginal, oral, or anal) increases your chance of contracting an STD or illness. While many STIs have no symptoms at all, some of them might resemble those of a urinary tract infection.

Bacteria that may infect the vaginal tract, for example, are the cause of chlamydia and gonorrhea. These STDs may also make urine painful or burning, much as UTIs do.

Research published in 2015 in the Journal of Clinical Microbiology found that STDs are often misdiagnosed as UTIs in women, despite the paucity of evidence in males. If you believe you could be carrying an STD, see your doctor. Antibiotics may be used to treat bacterial STDs like gonorrhea and chlamydia.

Chapter 5: Antibiotics, How to use them and their side effects

Bacteria entering your bladder, kidneys, or another section of your urinary system is the first sign of a urinary tract infection (UTI). The most effective approach to treat a UTI and get rid of symptoms like discomfort, burning, and a sudden desire to urinate is with antibiotics.

These drugs eliminate the germs that cause the ailment. It's crucial to take them exactly as directed by your doctor. If you don't get treatment, a small UTI might worsen into a dangerous kidney or blood infection.

The findings of your urine culture determine the antibiotic you get and how long you should take it.

Which drug will be most effective?
To determine if you have a UTI, your doctor will get a sample of your urine. The sort of bacteria you have will then be determined by the lab growing the germs in a plate for a few days. This is referred to as culture. Your doctor will

learn what kind of microorganisms caused your illness from this. To treat it before the culture is returned, they'll probably recommend one of the medicines listed below:

Amoxicillin/augmentin
Ceftriaxone (Rocephin) (Rocephin)
Cephalexin (Keflex) (Keflex)
Fosfomycin (Monurol), Ciprofloxacin (Cipro), and Levofloxacin (Levaquin)
Whether your infection is difficult or not will determine the medicine and dosage you get.

Your urinary tract is normal if it's "uncomplicated." "Complicated" refers to the presence of an illness or urinary tract issue. You could have a blockage like a kidney stone or an enlarged prostate, or you might have a narrowing of your ureters, which are the tubes that take urine from your kidneys to your bladder, or a constriction of the urethra, which carries pee from the bladder out of the body (in men). It's also conceivable that you have a bladder diverticulum or a urinary fistula.

Your doctor may suggest a greater dosage of antibiotics to treat a difficult illness. You may need to get high-dose antibiotics via an IV in a hospital or doctor's office if your UTI is severe or if the infection is in your kidneys.

When selecting an antibiotic, your doctor will also take into account the following:

Are you expecting?
You must be older than 65.
Do you have an allergy to any antibiotics?
Have antibiotic side effects ever occurred to you?

Trimethoprim is another widely used and efficient antibiotic for a UTI. There are 100mg and 200mg dosages of this UTI medication. Similar to Nitrofurantoin, Trimethoprim works by preventing bacterial development so that your immune system can combat the illness.

Treatment for cystitis that works well is trimethoprim. Trimethoprim may start working within a few hours, according to clinical investigations. Within 24 hours, it might reduce your UTI symptoms.

Trimethoprim dosage
With or without meals, trimethoprim pills should be swallowed whole. Urinary tract infections may be treated with it for both chronic and acute cases.

Trimethoprim is taken over three days. Two tablets every day, ideally taken at the same time each day to make remembering easier, should be taken. When your symptoms disappear, don't stop taking Trimethoprim. You can ensure that your urinary tract infection won't recur by completing the whole course.

If you miss a dosage, don't be concerned. Take a pill as soon as you remember to, please. If your next dosage is soon due, skip the missing dose.

To make up for a missing dosage, never take two pills at once.

Trimethoprim side effects
Trimethoprim comes with the same potential for adverse effects as any other UTI medication. Trimethoprim often causes the following adverse effects:

Rash skin
Diarrhea
Anemia
Throat pain
appetite loss
Additionally, disorientation, vertigo, jaundice, and mouth ulcers may occur in women using trimethoprim. After your cystitis treatment, most of these adverse effects will disappear. After finishing your Trimethoprim course, if you develop any of these symptoms, call your doctor right away.

If you are taking other medications, speak with your doctor. If you are nursing a baby, expecting a child, or have an allergy to any of the substances in Trimethoprim, your doctor may not advise you to take it.

Chapter 6:UTI in pregnancy

The common condition known as a urinary tract infection, or UTI, may often affect pregnant women. A UTI may be very harmful to a pregnant woman's health and the health of the baby while it is still growing.

The probable causes of a UTI during pregnancy are discussed in this article along with any associated dangers. The prevention and treatment of UTIs are other topics we cover.

Is it common?
Any portion of the urinary system, including the bladder and kidneys, may become infected; this is known as a UTI. Pregnant women often get UTIs, according to research. Trusted Source

Treatments
Women who are pregnant and exhibit any UTI symptoms should see their doctor. A UTI may have catastrophic consequences if left untreated.

If you get a UTI while pregnant, you may need to take antibiotics for three days. Trusted Source One of the following antibioticsTrusted Source may be prescribed by a physician:

amoxicillin
ampicillin\cephalosporins
nitrofurantoin\trimethoprim-sulfamethoxazole
The first trimester of pregnancy should be avoided by using trimethoprim-sulfamethoxazole and nitrofurantoin, according to the American College of Obstetricians and Gynecologists (ACOG). If a pregnant person takes these antibiotics at this point in the pregnancy, it might result in abnormal births.
In general, research demonstrates that trimethoprim-sulfamethoxazole and nitrofurantoin are safe to use throughout the second and third trimesters. But using either antibiotic in the last week before birth may make babies more susceptible to jaundice.

Women who get pregnant will require medical care if they acquire a kidney infection while pregnant. Antibiotics and intravenous fluids are part of this therapy.

It is quite improbable that a brief round of antibiotics can damage an unborn child. According to research, there is a huge difference between the dangers of not treating a UTI and the advantages of taking antibiotics.

Domestic remedies
The symptoms of a UTI should be seen by a doctor if the woman is pregnant. They may want to attempt the following at home in addition to medical care to hasten their recovery:

Water helps eliminate germs from the urinary system and dilutes urine, thus it should be consumed in large quantities.
Consuming cranberry juice: A 2012 assessment by Trusted Source found that cranberries contain substances that may help prevent germs from adhering to the lining of the urinary system. By doing so, the infection may be stopped and wiped out.

Having a bowel movement as soon as you feel the need can speed up the removal of germs from your urinary system.

the use of certain supplements According to research published in 2016 on Trusted Source, probiotics, cranberries, and vitamin C may be effective in treating women who get recurring UTIs.

Instead of using antibiotics, some women could choose the aforementioned therapies. But before doing so, they must always speak with their doctor. To assess the efficacy of home remedies and make sure a UTI does not become worse, a doctor will periodically check on a pregnant patient.

Complications

UTIs may have major negative effects on pregnancy if they are not treated. Problems might arise because of:

infected kidneys

birth defects and sepsis

Untreated UTIs may result in low birth weight in newborns, which is another risk factor.

Additional issues, such as the following, may result if a UTI progresses to the kidneys:

anemia

Hypertension, also known as high blood pressure

Hemolysis, low blood platelet count, thrombocytopenia, preeclampsia, red blood cell disintegration, and bacteremia are some examples of preeclampsia-related conditions.

respiratory distress syndrome with acute onset

Infection may sometimes spread to the newborn child, leading to a rare but serious problem. These risks may be avoided by going to prenatal UTI tests and seeking treatment once one develops.

Prevention

The probability of acquiring a UTI may be reduced by using the following advice:

Be sure to hydrate yourself.

Take cranberry supplements or unsweetened cranberry juice

Before and after having sex, cleanse the area surrounding the genitalia thoroughly, pee whenever the desire strikes, and at least every 2-3 hours.

Usually, early in their pregnancy, pregnant women will go to a screening to look for UTIs. These examinations are a critical first step in preventing or early identifying UTI infections.

UTIs are often seen, and some pregnant women may get them.

If a pregnant woman has UTI symptoms, she should see the doctor right once. A pregnant woman's health, as well as the health of the growing baby, might be seriously harmed by UTIs if left untreated. It is possible to avoid these consequences with prompt action.

Chapter 7: Home remedies to cure UTIS

Replacement of estrogen during menopause
Leave the baths alone.
Purchase a bidet and use it properly.
Maintaining the highest level of cleanliness and dryness is one of the best things you can do to avoid UTIs at home. It is recommended to wipe your body from front to back after urinating or having a bowel movement to promote good hygiene and prevent bacteria from entering the urethra and ascending the urinary tract.

2. Put on cotton underclothes
Make sure the urethra stays as clean and dry as possible to prevent bacterial entry by wearing undergarments made of natural fibers. Too-tight clothing can restrict airflow to the urethra. Without airflow, bacteria can get inside and breed in a setting that encourages the emergence of a UTI. Nylon and other synthetic fibers can hold moisture, which promotes the growth of bacteria when worn as clothing.

3. Be respectful

Although "good" bacteria are present and crucial for maintaining a healthy balance, the presence of any bacteria in the urinary tract does not necessarily indicate the presence of an infection. Douching can eradicate "good" bacteria as well as "bad" bacteria, altering the pH balance in your body. In the end, this might encourage the "bad" bacteria to proliferate. Through discharge, the vagina maintains itself. Use a pH-balanced formula like Summer's Eve if you still feel the need to wash down there.

4. Alternate soaps
Your UTIs might be caused by the bubble bath, body wash, and other cleaning supplies you use. Use fragrance- and dye-free formulas for sensitive skin.

5. Frequently swap out menstrual cups, tampons, or pads
Low-absorbency synthetic material pads put your vulva at risk of infection by exposing it to bacteria. It's critical to change your tampons frequently because using them can encourage bacteria to multiply more quickly. If used improperly, tampons and menstrual cups can

increase the likelihood that you will develop or worsen a UTI. Bacteria can spread to the bladder if something pushes against your urethra and traps your urine. Changing a menstrual cup's size or shape could help stop reoccurring UTIs.

6. Avoid spermicides.
A type of birth control called spermicide is inserted into the vagina before sex to kill sperm. Spermicides may irritate, removing protective barriers against bacterial invasion naturally present in the body (and ultimately infection). If you have a UTI, you should refrain from using spermicides. UTIs can also be avoided by urinating before and right after sex.

7. Add heat
Pubic pain or discomfort can result from having a UTI. It is simple to use heating pads or hot water bottles to relieve pain there. The pelvic region can benefit greatly from having heat applied for about 15 minutes. Any irritation or burning can be avoided by ensuring that the environment isn't too hot and that the skin isn't directly in contact with the heat source. Warm

baths may seem like a sensible way to ease UTI discomfort, but most medical experts advise against taking bubble baths. If you do take a bath, skip the soap and suds and just soak for a short while.

Drink water.
Drinking enough water is one of the greatest natural treatments for UTIs. Drinking plenty of water aids in the body's ability to flush away microorganisms. The typical healthy individual should have four to six glasses of water each day, according to Harvard Health.

Drink some cranberry juice.
A urinary tract infection may result from bacteria attaching to the cell walls of the urinary tract's cells. The active component of cranberry juice, proanthocyanidins, may help prevent UTIs by preventing germs from adhering to the walls of the urinary system. Cranberry juice lowers the number of UTIs a person may get over a year, according to research by the National Center for Biotechnology Information. The same effect is

achieved by several over-the-counter cranberry supplements in addition to cranberry juice.

The medical profession is quite divided on the topic of drinking unsweetened cranberry juice to treat UTIs. Some individuals may benefit from drinking the juice, while others may not. Whether or not cranberry juice is appropriate for treating UTIs is ultimately up to each patient.

10. Frequent urination
While suffering from a UTI, often urinating will aid in clearing germs from the urethra. The bladder may become more infected with urine-borne germs if the need to urinate is suppressed. Additionally, urinating before and after sexual activity will lessen the number of germs that enters the urethra.

Eat more garlic.
Garlic is widely renowned for its antibacterial and antifungal qualities, making garlic consumption a fantastic approach to strengthening your immune system. Allicin, one

of the chemicals in garlic, has antibacterial qualities that are efficient in eliminating E. coli.

12. Consume fewer sweets
According to Sarah Emily Sajdak, DAOM, an acupuncturist and traditional Chinese medicine practitioner in New York City, "Diet may be crucial in the prevention of UTI as it is caused by a bacterial infection." "Sugar is a favorite food of bacteria, so the more sugar you consume, the more you're feeding the illness,"

13. Add probiotics to your diet
Probiotics are dietary supplements that contain "good" bacteria and maintain a healthy immune system and gut. They may help treat and prevent recurring urinary tract infections and inhibit the growth of dangerous germs. For preventing UTIs in women, the probiotic lactobacillus has shown to be particularly helpful.

Probiotics may be bought in grocery shops or health food stores in a variety of forms. A healthcare expert should always be consulted if you're interested in taking them for UTIs and are unsure of which sort to obtain.

14. Use natural treatments
A plant known as ava Ursi possesses astringent, antiseptic, and anti-inflammatory effects. For both treating and preventing UTIs, avatars have shown to be useful. It is available at health food shops and has to be consumed as advised by a nutritionist or medical expert.

To prevent UTIs, Dr. Sajdak suggests the natural nutrients listed below in addition to uva ursi:

Cranberry tincture
Echinacea
Dandelion root with goldenseal
D-mannose
D-mannose is a kind of sugar that may prevent germs from adhering to the wall of the urinary system. According to some research, using D-mannose powder together with water may assist patients who regularly have UTIs avoid them.

Because they may interfere with other drugs you are taking for different reasons, all herbal supplements should be used in conjunction with a healthcare provider.

15. Use essential oils responsibly
The strong antimicrobial effects of oregano essential oil are widely established. Oregano oil has been found in studies to be quite successful in killing E. coli, although it should be emphasized that these tests are often in vitro, which means they are conducted in a lab setting using scientific methods rather than on infected patients. Due to their antibacterial qualities, lemongrass oil and clove oil may also be used as a home cure for UTIs; however, both have been tested against dangerous bacteria in studies comparable to those done with oregano oil.

Before employing essential oils as a therapy, caution should be taken. Ingesting these oils is not recommended, according to the National Association for Holistic Aromatherapy. Essential oils may instead be used topically in conjunction with a carrier oil or safely breathed via a diffuser.

Increase your vitamin C intake.

Theoretically, cranberry juice or dietary supplements containing cranberries might have comparable benefits to vitamin C, often known as ascorbic acid, in preventing UTIs. Large intakes of vitamin C, probably beyond the level attained from regular citrus fruit eating, may acidify the urine enough to prevent the development of germs, although the clinical evidence is few and sometimes inconsistent. Vitamin C probably won't be sufficient to get rid of a UTI on its own once you have one.

17. Think about changing your birth control.

The risk of UTIs has been connected to birth control techniques that include spermicides, as was previously mentioned. A source for recurring UTIs has also been shown to be various birth control techniques, such as intrauterine devices (IUDs). Consult your doctor if you have questions regarding birth control methods or believe your current contraceptive is to blame for your recurring urinary tract infections.

18. Estrogen treatment with menopause

A UTI may be more easily caused by bacteria entering the urinary system via thin, dry vaginal tissue that results from menopause's loss of estrogen. Lactobacilli, a "good" bacterium, have been proven to be less prevalent in the vagina as a result of this estrogen reduction. Topical estrogen replacement treatment may strengthen the urethra and promote the colonization of the vagina with beneficial microorganisms.

19. Avoid baths

Bath soaps are often used, however, they might irritate the urinary system and make it easier for germs to enter the body through the large intestine. If a person already has a UTI, having a bath with soap or even just sitting in hot water might make it worse.

20. Invest in a bidet

Because germs enter the urinary system via the urethra to cause UTIs, thorough washing is a vital step in UTI prevention. Using a bidet is one simple and practical technique to prevent feces from entering the urinary system and causing an infection.

Medicines for UTI

You could need an over-the-counter or prescription drug if home cures for your UTI aren't working. The director of men's health and urologic oncology at St. Francis Hospital on Long Island, David Samadi, MD, says over-the-counter nonsteroidal anti-inflammatory drugs, such as Advil, Motrin, and Naprosyn, "[give] symptom relief." There are other over-the-counter medicines, such as AZO Urinary Pain Relief or Uristat pills, whose primary component is phenazopyridine, which may assist lessen urinary tract irritation but won't address the underlying reason.

Antibiotics, which function by eradicating bacterial infections inside the body, are often used as part of prescription UTI therapy. Macrobid, Cipro, and Bactrim are common antibiotics used to treat UTIs.

The length of time someone may need to take antibiotics to treat a UTI varies. Even if you begin to feel better after taking an antibiotic, it is crucial to take the complete recommended dosage. Antibiotic resistance may result from early antibiotic course termination since not all of the bacteria may have been eradicated.

Antibiotic prophylaxis is a therapy approach where drugs prevent an infection rather than treat one, and it may be helpful for certain persons with recurrent UTIs. The same drugs that are used to treat UTIs may also be used to prevent them, however, the dosages will differ. On an individual basis, a healthcare expert may choose the right drug, dose, and form.

Chapter 8: Food to eat when you have UTIS

When you have a UTI, eating a balanced diet of nutritious foods is recommended. Prebiotic foods like onions and leeks are advised, along with cranberries and other fresh fruit, leafy green vegetables, and complex carbohydrates like whole grains, and leafy greens. A urinary tract infection should be cleared up by drinking plenty of water.

Eating for UTI
Let's look more closely at what I suggest you consume (and drink) when you have a urinary tract infection to understand how they might reduce symptoms and help avoid repeated UTIs:

1. Water It's necessary to drink adequate water before talking about meals.

According to scientific studies, consuming an additional 1.5 liters of water daily may help avoid UTIs. Water consumption may assist in flushing out an illness that is currently active.

My blog post, Does Drinking Lots of Water Help Cystitis?, has further information on how water aids UTIs.

(2) Cranberries
Thanks to a substance called D-mannose, cranberries, a well-known treatment for cystitis, also aid with the treatment of UTIs. Using the sugar molecule D-mannose, we can inhibit bacteria from adhering to the bladder wall and causing illness. To avoid any issues, the germs are then eliminated via our urine.

According to the Cochrane study's findings, cranberry extract may prevent urinary tract infections just as well as regular antibiotic usage does—without the latter's evident adverse effects.

With Echinacea and Uva-ursi as allies in the battle against the infection (see "What else may help when you have a UTI?" below), cranberry can be consumed or taken as a supplement. However, cranberry alone is not antibacterial, so it won't eradicate the illness. It may be worth attempting frequent cranberry consumption if you are prone to UTIs to avoid recurrence as well.

Watch the components in cranberry juice.
Check the components before drinking cranberry juice, which is often recommended as a fantastic beverage for UTIs. The illness may become worse since many cranberry juice products have a lot of added sugar.

3. Vegetables with leaves, green
Some excellent choices are broccoli, kale, and spinach. These are healthy for your whole body, brimming with essential nutrients, and they strengthen the immune system, which is essential for fending off harmful microorganisms.

4. Complex carbohydrates
However, not all carbohydrates are harmful—eating sugar might worsen a UTI. The white processed carbs that readily convert to sugar and are best avoided when you have a UTI are wonderful replacements for them since they are rich in fiber. Therefore, go for complex carbohydrates like whole grains, brown rice,

quinoa, beans, and starchy, root vegetables like potatoes, sweet potatoes, and parsnips instead of white bread, white spaghetti, or any cakes or pastries produced from white flour.

5. Frozen fruit
The essential vitamins, minerals, and other elements found in fruit support your whole body and boost your immune system. Sugar should be avoided while an infection is active, but it is still a nice sweet treat. Berries, which are lower in natural sugar than many other fruits and, in my view, are nature's sweet, make a terrific pick in general, but particularly when you're sick. All fruit contains natural sugars, but they are also rich in fiber, so choose whole fruits over fruit juice to ensure you get the advantages of fiber. Another smart move is to go for fresh fruit, preferably organic, rather than dried or canned.

• Prebiotics
For our microbiome to thrive and to maintain the proper balance of bacteria in our bodies, prebiotic foods are crucial. You may try prebiotic foods like apples, bananas, chicory,

Jerusalem artichokes, asparagus, garlic, onions, leeks, and leeks. In addition to this, you may consume Molkosan as a prebiotic beverage. L+ lactic acid, which is present in Molkosan, aids in fostering conditions that encourage the growth of good bacteria. Try the Molkosan Fruit Smoothie; it's wonderful, and you can combine it with your daily fruit and vegetable consumption. Note that vegetarians should avoid using Molkosan.

Uva-ursi

The herbal treatment for UTIs is ava-ursi, often known as bearberry. The urinary system immediately benefits from its quick action and antimicrobial activity. It doesn't cause thrush as antibiotics do. I advise keeping a bottle of uva-ursi tincture in the house to start taking at the first indication of illness since it is not a treatment that should be used long-term.

A substance known as arbutin seems to be responsible for the antibiotic effects, but as it is an extract of the whole plant, it also has a wide range of additional advantages in addition to acting as an antibiotic. It has astringent qualities and includes allantoin, which helps to soothe irritated and inflamed urinary channels.

Taking Uva-ursi for a week is advised, and after only 4 days of usage, symptoms should start to get better. You should see your doctor if your symptoms do not get better.

Echinacea
Several illnesses are treated using echinacea, a powerful antibacterial, and anti-inflammatory plant. Although it is popular as a treatment for colds and the flu, it is also useful in the management of urinary tract infections. Its antibacterial characteristics aid in the treatment of the illness, and its anti-inflammatory and immune-supportive effects will aid in preventing a recurrence.

Echinacea aids in immune system support, making it safe to use regularly to boost defenses against illness and stave against infection. I suggest increasing the frequency with which you take your Echinacea if you do begin to have infection-related symptoms. If you want to avoid infection, you may thus take it twice daily, and if you have any indications of an infection, you might take it five times daily.

Printed in Great Britain
by Amazon